THE

HOMEOPATHIC CO~~N~~

The Art of

INTERROGATION

includes
Pharmacopollaxy (Repetition of the Dose)

PIERRE SCHMIDT, M.D.

B. JAIN PUBLISHERS (P) LTD.
USA — EUROPE — INDIA

THE HOMEOPATHIC CONSULTATION – THE ART OF INTERROGATION

30th Impression: 2012

Published by Kuldeep Jain for

B. JAIN PUBLISHERS (P) LTD.
1921/10, Chuna Mandi, Paharganj, New Delhi 110 055 (INDIA)
Tel.: +91-11-4567 1000   Fax: +91-11-4567 1010
Email: info@bjain.com   Website: **www.bjain.com**

Printed in India by
J.J. Offset Printers

ISBN: 978-81-319-0026-0

THE HOMEOPATHIC CONSULTATION

THE ART OF INTERROGATION
Pierre Schmidt, M.D.

In choosing a subject, I have taken as my theme one after which so many beginners are sighing and to which I have, in fact, found really no sufficient and useful references in our homeopathic literature, however extensive.

On the other hand, I have learned through frequenting homeopathic dispensaries and hospitals how very rarely indeed did the practitioners really know how to apply exactly the teachings recommended by the Master, concerning the interrogation of the sick and homeopathic semiology; for, must we, after having listened to the patient, *direct* the interrogation in a given direction, either on the side of a presumed pathological diagnosis or toward a remedy suggested by the first recital made by the patient?

Or must we, against all we were taught in our studies, interrogate without any consideration whatever concerning either remedy or diagnosis, but make what we may call a *systematic* interrogation?

On the other hand, we all know the theoretical principles, but how many *apply* them *really fully?*

Is this question of interrogation simply a thing of theoretical interest or is it a matter of practical application?

Is it only a simple *vue de l'esprit?*

Is there real accord between theory and practice?

Now that homeopathy is developing and growing, and this especially in our Latin countries, France, Switzerland, Spain, Italy and South America, everywhere we hear young practitioners asking: *"But how to question the patient?", "What are the most useful and indispensable questions to ask?", What is the difference between the allopathic and the homeopathic consultation?"*

Theoretically speaking, we have certainly many precious *practical* suggestions concerning the questionnaire; *Hahnemann,* in his Organon, devotes more than sixty three paragraphs[1] where he speaks about the examination of the patient. *Von Boenninghausen* gives us excellent advice how to take the case. *Jahr* furnishes also a questionnaire, as well as others like *Mure, Perussel, Molinari, Landry, Claude,* then, more recently, *Close* and *Kent,* this last the only one who gives us a full questionnaire comprising more than thirty-two pages, entitled "What the Doctor Needs to Know in order to Make a Successful Prescription."

Finally, there is that of *Dr. Margaret Tyler.*

But, I bear in mind also the famous lecture of *Constantine Hering,* published in 1833 in the "Bibliothéque Homeopathique

---

1   §§ concerning the Interrogatoire, in S. Hahnemann's Organon, 5th French edition: 81-104, 139-141, 150-152, 167-171, 175, 177, 179m 181-184, 192, 198-200, 206-21, 216-220, 224, 240, 250, 253-256, 278

de Genève," in which he sets forth the theme how to trace the picture of the disease, his rules being summed up in four words:-

To listen, to write, to question, to co-ordinate.

It will not be my task this evening to develop theoretically these four precepts, my purpose being essentially to aim at the most useful and exclusively practical side of the question in general.

Consequently, I will not discuss the art of listening to the patient, not the best way to write one's observations, not yet the technique of the study and the co-ordination of the symptoms, or the question of the physical examination. We will take up this evening only with the third precept, the questioning, or examination, strictly speaking.

I will neither enter into long theoretical details about this question, nor propose to you the large ideal questionnaire, which would be the most complete and the most perfect. I have compiled a questionnaire of that kind after years of the study of my chronic cases, but as it covers more than thirty-six pages, I obviously cannot discuss it here.

The main purpose of the *allopathic consultation* is to establish a pathological diagnosis, to label the disease in the most modern nosological fashion. It is said and taught everywhere that without it no treatment should be attempted. For the old school, the investigation of objective pathological symptoms is absolutely essential. In this research, the interrogation plays rather a secondary role, examinations with a more or less complicated array of physical instruments or chemical analysis, but one moment of reflection only will show us that all these procedures only aim at determining the one or the many organs which are affected and to determine how far they are involved.

It is the hunting after end-products, after the results of disease.

If these results are not still manifested in a precise objective manner, and if the sick person suffers from functional troubles only, or even if these are not yet present and the patient is only complaining of subjective troubles, his case is arbitrarily decided. It is a nervous, psychic, imaginary case!

But in the *homeopathic consultation,* we are not at all satisfied with this investigation only. Its object is to establish how a given morbid affection has developed itself in a given subject, and to explore all the possible details of the evolution of such a disease in an individual, and how precisely this patient differs from all the others bearing the same diagnosis.

For example, an allopath, after having examined the throat of a patient, remarks that it is inflamed and covered with membranes from which he may take a part for laboratory examination. And, if the result of this examination be diphtheria, he will give an injection of serum. If it is said to be a simple infection, he will give an antiseptic gargle and a throat-paint.

If he has ten patients following the same diagnosis, the ten will be treated just the same.

(Which reminds me *á propos* of an amusing story a minister told me the other day. He used to wait outside the surgery for a certain doctor friend of his, to whom he ventured to make the remark it was always interesting to note how many of the patients came out with bottles of the same colored medicine. To this remark the only answer forthcoming was a look of rather confused embarrassment!)

On the contrary, a homeopath will inquire into all details which *differentiate* this *particular* patient from the ten others;

one would have the membranes on the right side, another on the left, and another on the velum of the palate. The appearance of the membrane may vary in color from green to yellow, black or white, according to the case; in others the consistency may, however, change, but especially interesting for the homeopath are the functional and subjective troubles of the patient. One may have burning or shooting pains, or may complain of dryness or rawness. Certain patients may alleviate their pain by drinking cold water or warm, or by eating solid food. The extension of the trouble from left to right or *vice versa,* or from the throat to the larynx or to the nose, all these differences may lead to a different homeopathic remedy.

Many details, forsooth seemingly of secondary importance, if not quite useless for the allopath, pathologically observed, which will however permit not only of precise diagnosis of the disease but especially the diagnosis of this given patient, and the homeopathic physician will be able to find his *own and particular* remedy, I mean the remedy adapting itself precisely to all the different characteristics and peculiarities of the case.

There exist more than fifty-six remedies for diphtheria, but there is a very small number corresponding really to all the symptoms pertaining to this particular patient. And this is where the task of the homeopath begins.

To know well how to observe, how exactly to interrogate, is the first step in this indispensable inquiry, and one which leads to the real remedy to be found.

This is, Mr. President, ladies and gentlemen, *why* I will take this evening in consideration the best questionnaire which will satisfy the following desiderata:-

1.   The minimum of the best questions to be asked from a patient when the time is limited.

2.　Most important and most necessary those questions to discover, not the pathological diagnosis but the therapeutic diagnosis, the general remedy corresponding to *the patient.*

3.　The questions to be asked, those for which we are sure to find a correspondence in our repertories and materia medica.

The interrogation, above all, must be *methodical.*

Of course, it goes without saying that the questions asked must be according to the purest principles of homeopathy, i.e.,

(a)　*To avoid direct questions,* for we know, if the patient answers with yes or no, the question is badly formed.

(b)　*Never to ask a question putting an answer, so to say, into the patient's mouth,* thus making sure not to bias his answer.

(c)　*To avoid all questions where the patient is obliged to choose* between two different alternatives, and respect the sacred rule to leave the patient always his own choice.

Of course, the physician must put himself, as Dr. Kent says, on the level of language comprehended by his patient. His attitude of seriousness and benevolence must help to stimulate the confidence of his patient.

On the other hand, he must know sufficiently his materia medica, so that his questions will be adapted to the comparison he will have to make further on. "Store up your materia medica so as to use it, and it will flow out as your language flows," in the well-known words of Kent.

The physician, by his manner of interrogation and general questions, must do everything not to determine, but to let the patient himself characterize the particular facts. "Say as little as you can, but keep the patient talking and help him to come close to the line and keep to the point."

Never allow yourself to hurry a patient, establish a fixed habit of examination that will stay with you. It is only when you keep up the most careful kind of work that you can set up your reputation and fulfill your highest use (Kent).

We can never sufficiently bear in mind how difficult is the art of interrogation, and all the importance that should be given to it. "One can learn very much from Socrates," observes Hering, "and the study of Plato is as important for us as Hippocrates."

To avoid all ambiguity, I will first give you some questions that in the course of your own practice you also will have frequently heart, demonstrating that many physicians show by the questions they ask that they have not grasped the thought of individualization. For example:

1. Direct questions:
   (a) Are you thirsty?
   (b) Are you irritable?
   (c) Have you got pain in the stomach?

2. Suggestive questions:
   (a) You do not stand the cold very well, do you?
   (b) You surely prefer to be consoled?
   (c) I suppose that you don't like too greasy and too rich food?

3. Questions where the patient must choose:
   (a) Do you prefer dry or wet weather?
   (b) Do you dream about sad or cheerful things?
   (c) Are your menses dark or light?

About the direct questions, it is quite frequent that a patient would say "Yes, I am thirsty," because he thinks about his morning coffee and his soup at noon but really does not drink anything besides. Or another would say "No," because he thinks that drinking tea, wine, lemon squash and soda do not mean thirst, this being reserved for ordinary water only.

Then, about the greasy or rich food, he will say that he does not like them because the doctor has said, "Too greasy." And about the menses, you will hear that they are dark, being really absolutely red, because a timid patient, having no choice between dark or light, will reply one or the other color in order to get rid of the question.

I think it is unnecessary to discuss every possible answer or error which will result by doing so, my purpose being to give you a list of questions avoiding precisely these errors, to present them to the criterium of your long experience and to submit it to your considered criticism. Of course, you are aware of the considerable advantage a beginner in homeopathy would have if he had not to wait for forty years, but be at once able to ask just the best and most exact questions aiming at a practical result, and to the answer of which he would be able to find a similar correspondence in our pathogenesis.

What would be really the use of a question about which we know no corresponding remedy? Of course, everything is useful, but I repeat that we are working here for practical results and not for theoretical purposes. We must adapt ourselves to the pathogenetic pictures of our materia medica, pictures which are very rich and precious.

To finish with this introduction, I cannot sufficiently criticize the method quoted in the book recently published, "La doctrine de l'Homeopathic francaise" where the physician, after a short physical examination, asks the patient about the symptoms of *Sepia* suggested by a yellow saddle he has observed on her nose, or those of *Lycopodium* on an irritable man complaining of his liver. This we may call the "torpedo method," in French "le torpillage." Because a patient has red lips you would ask him, "Have you got an empty, all-gone sensation in the stomach before noon?" "Do you not find it disagreeable to be in a standing position quite a while?" "Are you not obliged to put your feet out of the bed at night because they are burning." "You probably drink much and eat little, etc. ..."

Those two torpillage methods, the last one based only on direct and suggestive questions, the former one on two external symptoms, are most dangerous, especially for the beginner, as almost invariably a suggestionable patient impressed by the physician, will find present all the symptoms about which he is asked.

One may feel why such physicians do need to give drainage remedies in addition to four or five others, to be able to obtain something we will call a result.

It is *blunderbuss shooting,* ladies and gentlemen, for beginners of course a strong temptation, may be even an amusing method, even perhaps a necessary stage to something better. But the practitioner who is not afraid to work his materia medica, to study his repertories and to understand his Organon, will be able with a single shot—may I say, after the manner of my own fellow-countryman, Wilhelm Tell, "with one arrow"-to obtain the desired results, because his methodical and serious interrogation will give him a full picture of the disease, about which he will be able to consider what represents really the patient on the whole.

I will consider this matter later on.

We have classified our work in the following way:-

(a) What are the bases of interrogation? (That is, on what basis are the questions to be asked?)

(b) What is the best classification to adopt in interrogation?

(c) How to formulate the questions, in which way to be formulated?

(d) How are we to know if questions are well asked, and consequently well answered?

(e) I say again that I will not present here a *full* questionnaire, but the best and shortest questionnaire calculated to obtain the maximum results, the time being limited. And this will constitute the current questionnaire of the physician having at his disposal twenty to thirty minutes for the interrogation and examination of his patient.

A. WHAT ARE THE BASES OF INTERROGATION?

That is on what basis are the questions to be asked?

To this, I will answer that those questions must be ruled by the homeopathic semiology concerning the value of symptoms, considering always the patient in general, on the whole, to see the patient in his totality and not in his parts; not the disease, not the pathology, not the diagnosis, but the patient, living, feeling and thinking.

Of course, I will not consider the anamnesis, the part concerning hereditary and personal antecedents'; all references which are a part, evidently, of the interrogation of every patient, but not necessary to develop, as they offer absolutely no difficulties to the physician in comparison with the *active interrogation,* after the patient has exposed freely all his feelings and symptoms to his physician. Everyone should be very conversant with the masterly exposition given by Kent in his 23-26 lectures on his homeopathic philosophy.

B. WHAT CLASSIFICATION IS TO BE ADOPTED?

On one side, we have the counsel given by Hahnemann in his Organon, then the remarkable study of Kent in his 32-33 chapters concerning the value of symptoms, then the numerous classifications established by Grimmer, Gladwin, Green, Loos, Margaret Tyler, Del Mas, Stearns, to quote only those worthy of notice. It is impossible to discuss here every one of the proposed classifications, the broad lines of which, nevertheless, converge in the same direction: First mental symptoms, then general symptoms, then cravings and aversions, then sexual symptoms, including M.P., and finally sleep and dreams.

After this list come the local symptoms related to the organs.

But if, theoretically, this classification seems the most acceptable, practically, it is not so; and about this, experience has proved to me precious teachings.

In my early days of practice, I used always first to ask the mental symptoms, but very soon I came to see I was mistaken.

In fact, an unknown patient, knowing nothing whatever about homeopathy, feels hurt or resents this interrogation about his character when he comes to see you for a headache, a stye or an enlargement of his prostate. Very often too, he imagines that you are mistaking him for a mental case, and that you are making a disguised psychoanalysis. Very shortly, the physician sees by the patient's way of answering, his attitude and his look, the error he himself is committing.

On the other hand, to make the interrogation of the mental symptoms at the end of the questionnaire is also a mistake. Because then the patient is tired and has his mind on the fact that those questions have nothing to do with his disease, and have no relation whatever to it. Thus, he answers shortly, curtly, badly, manifesting very soon his impatience and his desire to get rid of the inquiry.

This is why experience has taught us that it is preferable to begin with the general symptoms, then to ask the questions related to the mentality, explaining rapidly to the patient the difference here between homeopathy and allopathy, the former being able to compare these symptoms with those obtained on the man in health, because of homeopathic experimentation only supposed to be made on the healthy man, and not, as the ordinary school does, on animals.

Then come the aversions and alimentary cravings, then the symptoms related to the sleep and dreams, and finally, for ladies, those concerning the menses, if it is possible to do so. The questions related to the sexual sphere can almost never be asked in the first consultation, especially in a short one. Sometimes it can be touched on when one is asked about heredity or personal history.

To close with, it is good to reconsider some of the symptoms predicated by the patient, especially those considered as rare, peculiar and striking, strange or uncommon, and to examine their modalities in order to see if really they deserve important consideration.

Here is the list of symptoms to be taken into consideration:

1. General symptoms

Horary aggravation, periodical season aggravation; by the weather; dry, wet, cold, hot, fog, sun, wind. Changes of weather: snow, storms; aggravation of temperature, draughts of air; tendency to take cold, desire or aggravation by the air; aggravation of position, by motion or by repose, riding in cars, sailing, prandial aggravation, appetite and thirst, aggravation by certain foods, wine, tobacco, drugs, vaccinations, cold or hot baths, seashore or mountain, clothing, wounds slow to heal, hemorrhages, fainting in rooms full of people, laterality (side affected).

2. Mental symptoms

The mental state of a human being can, on the whole, be resolved into four or five essential points; life or death, emotions, fears, irritability and sadness; and all these under hyper or hypo-manifestations.

The theoretical classification would be thus:

(a) Symptoms relating to the instinct of self-preservation (death, suicide, etc.).

(b) Ailments from grief, vexation, mortification, indignation, anger, bad news, disappointed love, etc.

(c) Fear, anguish, anxiety.

(d) Irritability, anger, violence, impatience, hastiness.

(e) Sadness, weeping, despair, effect of consolation.

Then, certain symptoms having no relation to these categories as, for example, jealousy, absent-mindedness, concentration, mania of scruples and as to trifles; modifications of the character before, during and after menses.

Instead of following this questionnaire in the above given order, it would be better to follow it in the reverse order; because one must begin with symptoms rather superficial and which do not go too deep into the mind of the patient, which latter is ultimately to be discovered.

For the practitioner who has his eyes open as well as his understanding, there are numerous mental symptoms that can be observed without saying one single word, as for example; timidity, loquacity, egotism, easily offended, embarrassed, exhilarated, easily startled, haughty, needless, suspicious, laughing immoderately, even some memory troubles, quiet or hurrying disposition, sighing patients, restless, weeping when speaking about certain symptoms; also, there are certain symptoms of which there is no need to ask the patient because he will tell them himself, either because he came for this purpose, or suffers really very much on account of it. Very often, also, friends or relatives may have written of those symptoms to you before the consultation, if they are sufficiently striking, as, for example, the refusal to eat, the desire to escape, sometimes even fear of suicide, etc.

3.   Aversions and Alimentary Cravings

    (a)   Sweets, pastry, delicacies.

    (b)   Salty things.

    (c)   Sour, strong and spiced food.

    (d)   Greasy and rich foods, butter.

    (e)   Bread, fruits, fish, meat.

    (f)   Milk, coffee, wine, beer.

    (g)   State of thirst and appetite.

4.   Sleep and Dreams

    (a)   Position of the body, head and extremities during sleep.

    (b)   What the patient is doing during sleep; laughs, starts, talks, shrieks, weeps, is afraid, grinds his teeth, keeps eyes or mouth open, etc.

    (c)   Quality of the sleep: hours and causes of waking, of sleeplessness and sleepiness.

    (d)   All about dreams.

5. Symptoms concerning the menses and the sexual sphere

(a) M.P. too late, duration, abundance, color, quality, consistence, more day or night, influence of the character or other particular symptoms before, during and after the M.P., shortly all about what we call the "Molimen."

6. Rare, strange and peculiar symptoms

Uncommon symptoms indicated by the patient, with their modalities and related phenomena and the making more precise of the main symptoms for which the consultation was made.

Now, let us see this theoretical list of questions realized in a practical way, according to the Hahnemannian principles. I have just purposely chosen questions corresponding to repertory rubrics, which are of a middle size and containing, when possible, two or three degrees of remedies (italic and heavy type) and avoided the longer paragraphs like those of sadness, night aggravation, thirst, etc., which contain almost all the remedies.

C. HOW TO FORMULATE THE QUESTIONS

It is not a bad procedure to say to the patient at this time: "I have listened to you until now without interrupting you, now we will change the role, and please don't be astonished if I seemingly stop you while answering, to ask you the next question, because this will mean that the answer I was waiting for is obtained. Do not believe that by so doing, I under-estimate your answer, but this only signifies that a longer explanation will bring neither useful nor new details in the case."

General Symptom

1. At what time in the twenty-four hours do you feel worst?

2. In which season do you feel less well?

3. How do you stand the cold, hot, dry, wet weather?

4. How does fog affect you?

5. What do you feel when exposed to the sun?

6. How does change of weather affect you?

7. What about snow?

8. What kind of climate is objectionable to you, and where would you choose to spend your vacation?

9. How do you feel before, during and after a storm?

10. What are your reactions to north wind, south wind, to the wind in general?

11. What about draughts of air and changes of temperature?

12. What about warmth in general, warmth of the bed, of the room, of the stove?

13. How do you react to extremes of temperature?

14. What difference do you make in your clothing in winter?

15. What about taking colds in winter and in other seasons?

16. How do you keep your window at night?

17. What position do you like best—sitting, standing, lying?

18. How do you feel standing a while, or kneeling in church?

    You remark that this question of the standing position comes again. You will find this way of repeating it is intentional here and there in the questionnaire. It is a very useful and necessary procedure for verification.

19. What sports do you engage in?

20. What about riding in cars or sailing?

21. How do you feel before, during and after meals?

22. What about your appetite, how do you feel if you go without a meal?

It will be often answered to you: "I can easily go without a meal but I never can stand a big dinner or banquet." A question that you did not ask, but which demonstrates that the question was well formulated as it made the patient talk and left him his own choice.

23. What quantity and what do you drink? What about thirst?

24. What are the foods that make you sick, and why?

(If the patient does not answer after a while, just ask looking closely at him: sweets, salty things, sour, greasy food, eggs, meat, pork, bread, butter, vegetables, cabbages, onions, fruits?)

25. What about wine, beer, coffee, tea, milk, vinegar?

26. How much do you smoke in a day, and how do you feel after smoking?

27. What are the drugs to which you are very sensitive or which make you sick?

28. What are the vaccinations you have had, and the results from them?

29. What about cold or warm baths, sea baths?

30. How do you feel at the seaside, or on high mountains?

31. How do collars, belts and tight clothing affect you?

32. How long are your wounds in healing, how long in bleeding?

33. In what circumstances have you felt like fainting.

Mental Symptoms

34. What are the greatest griefs that you have gone through in your life?

    (Quite often the patient will lower the head and look quite moved, and a kind word of the doctor will be needed. It is why, as soon as the extra-version or self-expression has been made, this following question will make the patient look at you again in an astonished way, and sometimes with a happy smile).

35. What are the greatest joys you have had in life?

    These two questions are very important and, when asked at the right moment, will pave the way for the coming questions.

36. At what time in the twenty-four hours do you feel in the blues, depressed, sad, pessimistic?

37. How do you stand worries?

38. On what occasions do you weep?

    (If the patient cannot answer, we will just ask – not losing for one second his expression – music, at reproaches, at which time of the day? Certain people can refrain from weeping, some others cannot).

39. What effect has consolation on you?

    (If the answer is, "It depends by whom," you may say; "just by people you like," because very often people say they do not like to be comforted because they think of members of their family they hate.)

40. On what occasions do you feel despair?

41. In what circumstances have you ever felt jealous?

42. When and on what occasions do you feel frightened or anxious?

(If the patient does not answer, ask, some people are afraid of the night, of darkness, to be alone, of robbers, of certain animals, of death, of certain diseases, of ghosts, to lose their reason, of noises at night, of poverty, of storm, of water. According to the way of answering, you will at once see the real fears, and be able to discriminate those which are not to be taken into consideration.)

43. How do you feel in a room full of people, at church, at a lecture?

44. Do you go red or white when you are angry, and how do you feel afterwards?

45. How do you stand waiting?

(If he does not answer, just question him about impatience.)

46. How rapidly do you walk, eat, talk, write?

47. What have been the complaints or effects following chagrin, grief, disappointed love, vexation, mortification, indignation, bad news, fright?

48. In time of depression, how do you look at death?

(Certain patients have presentiments of death, thoughts of death, even desire to die; others have tendencies or desires of suicide, some would be courageous enough to do it, others are afraid, in spite of desiring it.)

49. Tell me all about over-conscientiousness and over scrupulousness, about trifles; some people do not care about too much details and too much order.

50. What about your character before, during and after menses?

During all these questions, the physician must by kind words put his patient at ease, but must watch him very closely, without the patient's noticing it.

Food Cravings and Aversions

(a) What is the kind of food for which you have a marked craving or aversion, or what are those that make you sick or you cannot eat?

Here also, it is very important to watch very carefully the expression of the patient, because it is very easy to read on the face by observing the corners of the mouth coming down if the patient is disgusted, or on the contrary coming up with big shining eyes if the craving or a strong alimentary attraction is felt. Then, one can add, for example:

(b) What about pastry and sweets?

(c) What about sour or spiced food?

(d) What about rich or greasy food?

(e) How much salt do you need for your taste?

(f) What about thirst and what do you drink?

Coffee, wine, beer, etc…

Of course, all those questions have been already asked in the beginning of the questionnaire, but by asking them again, you are able, by doing some cross questioning, to determine if they have been answered well the first time or not.

Sleep

(a) In which position do you sleep, and since when that position? Where do you put your arms, and how do you like to have your head?

(b) What are you doing during sleep?

(If the patient does not answer, you add, some people speak, laugh, shriek, weep, are restless, and are afraid, grind their teeth, have their mouth or their eyes open.)

(c)   At what time do you wake up, or when are you sleepy? What makes you restless or sleepy?

(d)   What about dreams?

For Ladies - Menses

(a)   At what age did they begin?

(b)   How frequently do they come?

(c)   What about their duration, abundance, color, odor, what about clots, etc.

(d)   At what time in the twenty-four hours do they flow most?

(e)   How do you feel before, during and after menses?

Retaking the Case

It is necessary to take through again in the symptoms told by the patient, those which were strange, rare and peculiar, for example, sensation of a nail in the head; feeling of a string drawing back the eyeballs, feeling of a lump in the throat, a griping feeling in the heart, feeling of a constriction like a bandage around the knees.

All those must be carefully noted, in order that the physician may ascertain himself that there are no occasional causes provoking them.

Then, about some other outstanding symptoms; it is important to take the modalities concerning the aggravation or amelioration by motion, repose, heat or cold, in or outdoors, position, eating, pressure, etc.

D. HOW NOW, TO KNOW IF THE QUESTIONS ARE WELL ASKED AND, CONSEQUENTLY, WELL ANSWERED?

There are two ways of knowing:

1. During all the interrogation, the physician must carefully watch his patient and observe the way he answers. As in La Fontaine's fable, the "rampage" must accord with the "plumage," i.e., the intonation of his voice, the play and expression of his physiognomy, especially in mouth and eyes, must be carefully observed and grasped.

   A patient who says, "Yes, I like meat, but I don't drink milk with pleasure" without change of expression indicates no symptom at all. But if he says, "Oh, I cannot do without meat, and I hate milk," saying this with a happy face and an enlargement of the eyes regarding meat, but regarding milk with a wry face, while turning the head to the side, you then know you have good symptoms.

   Of course, beside the question of useful and useless symptoms, in the useful symptoms there is still a gradation. There are very marked and also less important ones, but this comes into consideration only if we have quite a number of them. On the occasion of the first interrogation, we will have little to do with this consideration, and be happy to have only a sufficient number of symptoms.

2. During the interrogation, the physician is carefully noting in writing all the answers of his patient. He underlines or marks with a cross those which are of importance to be further cross-questioned or verified in order to be assured that the patient has *really well understood and well answered* the question.

   This is to put it to the proof.

Then, we have seriously to consider making quite a number of cross-questions. For example:

If the patient has told you that he feels worse after meals, you may ask him, "If you have an important matter to decide or a delicate letter to write, or some important call to make, would you do it at 2 p.m.?"

If he told you that he was sleeping with his hands outstretched over his head, you may ask him, "During sleep, would the warmth of the bed clothes cause your hands to perspire?"

If he tells you that he hates greasy food, "Do you prefer the fish with sauce, or fried, or in black butter? And how do you like bacon?"

If he says that pity or consolation aggravate him, ask him if he has a friend to whom he gives his confidence when he is worried.

Should he assert he is never angry, ask him if he is red or white when angry. Very often, the answer will be, "Red, but it passes rapidly away."

To be certain that some symptoms are to be retained and good, these few above-mentioned examples will suggest you to know how to ask these questions.

Very often, a patient says that he is very impatient, but you can observe that, after having sat for half an hour in your waiting room, he walks calmly into your consulting room and responds most calmly to your questions.

Another will tell you that he is even-tempered, but you learn that he is divorced or that he has left his family because of incompatibility of character.

If one, two or more remedies come to your mind after such an examination, and you are hesitating between this one and the other, that is the only occasion where one is authorized to ask some questions, always based on the same principles, but relative to the symptoms characteristic of the remedy suggested, always, obviously trying to avoid direct questions and the torpillage methods already referred to. Very often, it would be better and more prudent to give S.L., rather than to administer a remedy that is not absolutely indicated, about which we are not sure, and have the courage to await the second consultation in order to complete the picture of the disease.

The purpose of this paper is not to examine what is to be done with the symptoms thus obtained or how to classify them, or how to find the corresponding simillimum in the materia medica. If one follows this classification, the second part of the work, the grading and classification of symptoms would be nearly completed for the physician.

I observed that certain questions are always answered in the same way, by almost everybody, and consequently I consider those bad questions. Sometimes, too, the patient indicates some symptoms which seems very important, and which he has not in reality. He will inform you that he has some abilities or qualities, and you observe just the contrary.

That is why I think that a questionnaire established with method and reflection is indispensable, and that is why I have submitted it to you this evening, desiring to know your own experiences and what are the questions to suppress, to develop, or in which order to ask them.

I always try to practice the advice of my esteemed teacher, Dr. Austin of New York, who told me that a good physician should be able in the first consultation to make his patient laugh or cry, and so doing, he was assured that the contact was made, as he was able to put in vibration the living human being who was asking for *help*.

If, in the allopathic consultation, as we were told and taught in our allopathic studies, one must not believe his patient, must ask the fewest questions possible and believe only what could be observed by the physician himself, this is quite different in homeopathic consultation, because the homeopathic physician must do his best to create around him an atmosphere of confidence and benevolence, and try to comprehend especially the human being who comes to be helped. The most important task in homeopathy is to individualize and to discriminate, but individualization and comparison are inseparable, and there is a difference in the nature of things most similar, a point that must be carefully considered.

The substitution of one remedy for another cannot be thought of or entertained in homeopathy, and Kent repeats what Hahnemann says: "In homeopathy, medicines can never replace each other nor be as good as another."

One cannot repeat enough that if the first examination is well established, well made, well realized and well interpreted, the search after the remedy will be but a sole thing, and if the case has been well taken and the remedy based really on the most important symptoms, all this being rightly done at the first consultation, the work for the physician will be considerably easier because he has found the thread and has only to follow it. On the contrary, this treatment based on local examination or insufficient interrogation will oblige you to zigzag perpetually and, instead of feeling your prescription based on an edifice with large foundations, you have the impression of a cork floating on the ocean.

Nothing is more culpable than to say, "*Thuja* is your remedy, because I see that you are perspiring on your upper lip!" (the repertory has seven remedies for this sole symptom) or, "You are *Lachesis* because your lips are blue and varnished," or "You are a case of *Condurango* because you have cracks in the corners of the mouth."

If I speak here about *Condurango*, it is to confess my *mea culpa*.

Eleven years ago, when I came to the London Homeopathic Hospital for the first time, I was very kindly authorized to follow the visiting physician round the wards. It happened to be the day of Sir J. Weir. I did not know him; was he a good or a bad homeopath? Did he know anything about it? Very soon I would be able to decide for myself.

Just arrived from Geneva, after having studied homeopathy in the "Catechism of Dr. Dewey" and the "Organon of Hahnemann," I thought I had the whole of homeopathic knowledge and wisdom. This was all the more so as I had already treated some cases with success, having received the benefit of the experience of a physician who had given me advice in some rather more difficult cases.

After having seen some patients, we stopped before a bed where a new patient had just come, and I still remember and can see Sir John Weir, his head bending towards the patient, asking innumerable questions. As soon as one was answered, another was quickly formulated.

In the beginning, this impressed me, but I rapidly saw that the patient had quite a red patch on the right corner of her mouth with a deep crack.

This reminded me of a similar case where I was puzzled about the indicated remedy and where a homeopath told me: "It is a plain *Condurango* case." As soon as Sir John Weir was through, feeling the marked superiority of my knowledge and seeing that after this long and elaborate interrogation he had not mentioned any remedy, I told him, "Don't you see that it is a plain case of *Condurango*?" Very kindly he turned his head and, without irony or reproach but bowing his head, he said very politely: "I thank you, Sir; we will discuss this later on." Everyone around turned on me with an appreciative look at my cleverness.

After the visit we went down, and I then had my bad quarter of an hour *(mauvais quart d'heure)* – my cold douche.

"Well," said Sir John, "why is it a case of *Condurango*? Simply because of this crack in the corners of the mouth." "But," said he, "what about all her other symptoms?"

"Oh, they are of no importance. If you look carefully at her tongue, you surely will find some denuded areas and also some gastric symptoms and this will confirm and prove your *Condurango*.*"

"Well, well," said Sir John, "let us see." He simply opened a large book like the Bible and asked me if I knew it. "No." said I; "have homeopaths written such large books?" "It is the Repertory of Kent," he replied, "and see here that twenty-two remedies stand beside *Condurango* for cracks in the mouth."

With kindness but persuasion he very rapidly pulled to pieces all my illusions and my assurance.

He convinced me that this was a case of *Sepia*, explaining to me patiently why among the many symptoms there was a discrimination to be made, how interesting and of the utmost importance a hierarchic classification was to be made and that rules and principles were to be followed for such a study, why *Sepia* was the remedy for this patient and not *Condurango*. It was the most beautiful lesson in modesty that I ever received.

I shriveled inside and perspired outside. I had brilliantly demonstrated my deep and profound ignorance and unveiled my incapacity. But I probably was still not baptized, as when I went to New York, Dr. Austin at my first interview asked me which were the homeopathic remedies for rheumatism and, after I had spoken about *Rhus-tox.* and *Bryonia,* he gave me the last blow to my knowledge, saying simply:

"Well, my brother, I think it will be necessary to study homeopathy."

Thus, I learned to live out this famous sentence of the philosopher: "All I know is, that I know, I know nothing!"

In the same way, if your interrogation is not based on the essential principles of the homeopathic doctrine, if you are led by your caprice or fancy only and interrogate just about the symptoms the patient is complaining of, you will make only patchwork and end in failure. This failure would only demonstrate your own ignorance.

If a patient presents herself to you with varicose veins and pain in the lower limbs and you give her *Fluoric acid, Calcarea fluorica* or *Hamamelis,* you will have treated only the vascular walls, but not all the varicose patient. This is only a travesty of homeopathy. It is the application of a remedy to a diagnosis, it is allopathic prescribing with homeopathic remedies.

If the patient adds that she has agglutinated eyes in the morning and that her hairs are falling away, you would think at once of *Graphites* or *Sulphur.* But if she adds still further that she is bleeding from the nose, is very thirsty and craving acids, you will turn your preference to *Phosphorus*. You may then ask if she feels an empty sensation at the stomach and suffers from heartburn, in consultation, she will confess that she is suffering from a very distended abdomen, that she is constipated, her sleep is unrefreshing, liking better to be outdoors, so you will say: "Now it is clear, it is *Lycopodium*," and so on, continually. Like the wandering Jew, you err in this labyrinth, losing your head and often your patience. Why? Because you have not made a systematic and methodical examination, established according to the rules formerly given.

If you go through the short, but quite full interrogation given before, you will learn that this patient has her menses more at night, and the study of this case will show you very rapidly and clear as water that only one remedy covers all these symptoms, except the varicose veins, it is true, and here the remedy is *Magnesia carbonica*, not for or against the varicose veins, but *for* the patient who will be cured, and the varicose veins besides.

I described this case *en passant* because it is precisely one of my successful cures of varicose veins. The patient was cured, her varicose veins disappeared, like all the other miseries: gastritis, epistaxis, etc.... You will not be astonished to know that this depressed patient is now cheerful and enterprising, and that the beautiful mass of her black hair justifies her legitimate pride.

The homeopathic interrogatory includes, as you see, rules to be followed and a technique to be observed.

This interrogation, made according to the suggestions given in the beginning of this paper, will permit of the physician individualizing his case after an interrogation well made, a precious stone in the walls of the therapeutic edifice.

Physicians cannot sufficiently avoid every partiality to influence the patient from whom he has to elicit symptoms, related to remedies of which he may think, and which come to his mind by the first answer given by the patient. "He has a key to the patient and examines the patient by the key, that is, as Kent says, by the drug, a bad practice and never to be resorted to except as a dernier resort and in stupid patient." Doing so, we are on the wrong track which will end only in pitfalls.

The more objective the symptoms, the more they are to be observed of the patient dead, in his coffin, the less value have they. On the contrary, the more they express the living, feeling, thinking human being, the more important they are.

To establish a questionnaire really useful to the busy physician for his daily practice, a questionnaire based on the pure doctrine of homeopathy, such has been my purpose this evening. My endeavour will be more than fully rewarded and compensated if I may be told what further to add, to take away, to modify or to render it more perfect.

Knowing the valued knowledge and opinions of the members of your society, I submit this most important question to your esteemed consideration.

The Homeopathic Recorder

PHARMACOPOLLAXY

This term is derived from the union of two Greek words *Pharmacon*, meaning remedy, and *pollaxis*, meaning many times, and means really, *'the repetition of the remedy.'*

It is not my purpose to develop here all the modalities concerning this controversed question, which has been also applied so differently, but to place myself to a higher point of view, and here I will put the question in those terms: What do we mean by the repetition of the remedy?

At first, it seems that this question is very simple and clear, nevertheless it has been so much obscured that one could find commonly in our school this too frequently used expression: *the repetition of the dose*. What signifies this locution? Dr. Jahr asserts that the administration of the remedy in watery solution does not constitute a repetition, of the dose. This is really the way to darken and complicate this subject. No, the fact of giving a remedy in a successive manner, no matter in which form, is not – homeopathically speaking—a fraction of this remedy, but really the repetition of the very remedy each time it is given.

This is why Hahnemann, in his first volume of the Materia Medica, in the French edition, stipulates in his eighth paragraph this very question, writing as the title of his chapter:

On the repetition of homeopathic medicaments.

The master could have said in this title: the repetition of the doses, if it had been his opinion. So, it seems clear that in his very thoughts, every time one is repeating a dose he is repeating the remedy and the *whole remedy*. This chapter begins with those words:

"In the Organon I have insisted on the necessity never to give at the same time but one single dose of a well chosen homeopathic medicament, and to let it have all the necessary time to develop its action."

Evidently here the words *single dose* signify a remedy given at one single time. Of course, if one repeats many times this dose, he repeats as frequently this remedy.

One gives each time what represents the whole of the remedy, and not a fraction of it. Moreover in the chronic diseases, when we repeat the "dose at long intervals, do we not give each time the remedy?

A little further in this chapter, Hahnemann says again:

"Thus, a primitive psoric eruption, on a patient which is not too much weakened, even if it has invaded the whole body, can be perfectly cured through one dose of Tincture Sulph. Xe (30th dil.) repeated every seven days in the course of ten to twelve weeks" (consequently with 10 to 12 globules).

This term *consequently*, in this parenthesis explains the thought of the master. Those who know and understand the writings of Hahnemann, know very well that for him each globule contains the remedy on the whole.

Here are again some very intelligible and explicit words about it:

"But if the physician has to give a same substance more than one time, what is indispensable in order to cure serious

chronic diseases, he should be careful to change each time the degree of dynamization, even very slightly, the vital force of the patient can support the same medicament even at short intervals an incredible number of times, one after another and this with the greatest success... "

Dr. Mure, in his *Doctrine of Rio,* is still clearer and more precise:

"One single globule dissolved in a glass of water and taken by spoonfuls, every twelve hours, constitutes as many doses as the number of spoonfuls taken."

In homeopathy nothing will increase the energy or intensity and the rapidity of actions of remedy by augmenting or multiplying its quantity.

At last, the spirit of our doctrine teaches us that in the series of potentization, each vial contains the remedy on the whole, and every one of the hundred drops of the vial contains the whole remedy, to this degree in the series.

We must never forget, as has been said already by Granier, a French homeopath, that our remedies are not the so-called infinitely smalls, and we must forever let this faulty locution disappear. Our remedies are dynamic agents, like the miasms, and ought to be called *miasmoid.* The presence of matter is here absolutely out of the question.

The doctrine of the repetition of the remedy is virtually contained in the following sentence taken from the writings of our master:

"It goes without saying that before the physician permits himself to repeat the dose of a medicament, he should be absolutely convinced that it was perfectly well chosen and homeopathically indicated."

One should never say *repetition of the dose,* but we should say, *repetition of the remedy.*

Every time Hahnemann speaks about the repetition of the doses, it is only a negligence of language, also every time he speaks of a *medicament* instead of a remedy. In fact, the medicament, through experimentation or proving produces the phenomena and pertains to pathology. The *remedy* on the contrary, through experiments, neutralizes the symptoms and pertains to nosology. To the old school, the remedy is a remedy *a priori,* without anything prior to it, but for our school, the remedy is considered as such only *a posteriori,* having as its starting point its study on the healthy man. To the homeopathic school, every remedy before its application must have been a medicament.

Of course, it is not our purpose on this occasion to give all the wise advices resulting from the vast experience of the master concerning the repetition of the remedy. For those who have taken the time to read carefully and to study the preface of the *Chronic Diseases,* the *Lesser Writings,* the preface of each volume of the *Materia Medica Pura* and the *Organon,* it is very clear to understand that our master has said almost everything touching the pharmacopollaxy.

In conclusion, we can say that:

1.   The ideal to be realized, as Hahnemann said, would be to treat every disease with *one single remedy* and one single dose. Of course, this supposes a very careful study and quite perfect correspondence of the remedy to the sick patient.

2.   The repetition of the remedy requires positive and strong reasons. The principal reason of the repetition of the remedy must be based on the vital reception, on the individual reaction which is called susceptibility of the patient, the

less sensitive is the patient, the more one is permitted to repeat.

3. The repetition of the remedy depends also on the nature of the remedy.

4. The repetition of the remedy must be submitted to the nature of the disease as well as to the nature of the remedy.

5. The repetition of the remedy depends on the duration of the action of the remedy. Everyone knows that *Calcarea* has a longer duration of action than *Ignatia*.

6. The repetition of the remedy depends on its dynamization (potency).

7. In chronic diseases, one must be very careful with the repetition and you will never regret to repeat at long intervals, rather than too shortly.

8 In acute diseases, experience teaches us that the repetition can be done most frequently. Nevertheless many beautiful cases have been cured with one single dose or a few doses. (High fever, great pain, great fear, strong fits of anger or emotional excitement shorten the action of a remedy and indicate repetition.)

9. Hahnemann has repeated:

"And nothing is more guilty than to repeat blindly and routinarily a remedy, one must be guided always by the reaction of the patient and observe carefully the direction and course of the symptoms, ... One must be very careful not to use prevision in the indications of the homeopathic remedies and should always base his prescription on the actual totality: it is impossible to prescribe different remedies in advance, either mixed or alternated, for this is a practice absolutely aside from the principles of our doctrine, it is only empiricism, and the work of the most

*pitiful routine. ... The homeopathic physician ought to
examine the symptoms every time he prescribes; otherwise
he cannot know whether the same remedy is indicated a
second time, or whether a medicine is at all appropriate."*

10. The most important thing about the repetition is the careful
observation of the patient and disease, so as to ascertain
precisely which is which, pertains to the one or the other.
More harm has been done by repeating doses than by giving
too rarely a remedy. One is amazed to observe all the
possibilities of the single dose when the field for its action
is free and no interference perturbs itpossibilities. There
are great forces that we still do not dream of, and one
impulse, as small as it seems to be, has its place in the right
moment, according to the law of nature, and can bring
results which are really extraordinary.

11. We must add, as Hahnemann says; *There are exceptions to
the rule, which it is, however, not the business of every
beginner to discover.*

12. The repetition of the remedy is one of the most important
things after the careful selection of the remedy and its
careful prescription. It needs not a worried, nervous or
restless physician; but very careful observation, patience,
knowledge and also courage are the qualities required for
a master in prescribing. The homeopathic physician is
surely the one who must be most careful about this question
and who is able to learn very much if he knows how to
watch and wait, after having given his remedy. No routine
must preside to the decision of such a homeopathician, for
he must act only according to law and principles, as Kent
beautifully describes it in his chapter concerning the second
prescription:

Hahnemann, Chronic Diseases, p. 160, loc. cit.

*"No repetition is to be considered unless the record has
been again fully studied, unless the first examination, and all
the things that have since arisen, have been carefully restudied
that they may be brought again to the mind of the physician."**

The Homeopathic Recorder

---

*   *Chronic Diseases*, trad. Hempel, 1845, Vol. I, p. 161.